TABLE

Introduction

Chapter 1: Understanding Anti-Inflammatory Diet

Chapter 2: The Manuscript

Chapter 3: Foods to Avoid

Chapter 4: Anti-Inflammatory Foods

Chapter 5: Implementing an Anti-Inflammatory Diet

Chapter 6: Recipes

Conclusion

Will you review this book?

FREE Bonus – My Gift for You!!!

More Books You Might Like

INTRODUCTION

I want to thank you and congratulate you for downloading the book, "Anti-Inflammatory Diet".

This book contains proven steps and strategies for beginners to smoothly incorporate an Anti-Inflammatory diet into their everyday life and reap the long-term health benefits associated with it.

The 21st-century healthy lifestyle movement is arguably the most dominant trend that the world has ever experienced. This phenomenon has swept across the globe, leaving no stones unturned. Regardless of the country or continent, the effects of this healthier living campaign are evident. Given its broad definition, this movement can present itself in many forms and it can be hard to keep track of all its latest developments.

In the early stages, health activists vigorously promoted the importance of regular physical activities as part of the criteria towards sustaining a prolonged carefree life. Fueled by the insatiable desire of the global population, these advocates continually explored the possibilities of other methods in order to further the healthy lifestyle campaign. This paved the way for doctors to introduce the notion of healthier dietary plans to aid in the universal pursuit of maximizing health condition.

The distinct advantage of prescribing to healthier food choices lies in its ability to be modified and customized to cater to specific individuals with unique requirements. Its all-encompassing benefits can be utilized to assist people with various objectives ranging from achieving weight loss targets to countering the effects of aging. Due to the overwhelming popularity of this approach, the internet is awash with dietary plans formulated by health experts that claim to effectively extend life expectancy.

As laymen continue to yearn for the mystical fountain of youth or immortality pill, health professionals, and scientists are putting in the extra effort to combine medical treatments and scientific discoveries to derive at the next best alternative towards prolonging the human lifespan. With technological advancement at its peak, health experts are constantly gaining new insights into the association between individual diet, genes, and health. One of the major breakthroughs in this area is the establishment of the fact that diets can alter the expression of the human genes. This groundbreaking revelation gives rise to the possibility that the best method to cure certain illnesses or diseases can be found in the kitchen, rather than in medicine cabinets.

Based on the fundamentals of this concept, doctors developed the anti-inflammatory diet to combat the undeniable correlation between chronic inflammation and certain illnesses. Credible research and studies have shown that many illnesses, such as Alzheimer's disease, Parkinson's disease, various cardiovascular diseases and even some form of cancers, can be traced back to chronic inflammation.

Inflammation can be defined as local redness, pain, heat or swelling experienced by the body. It is responsible for causing a sprained ankle to swell and an infection to bring on a fever. Inflammation is a biochemical reaction triggered by the wound healing coagulation structure. It is an internal alarm system and the cornerstone of the healing process as it alerts the immune system to channel more nourishment to the affected area. The immune system then attacks anything foreign, such as chemicals, plant pollens or invading microbes.

While this process between inflammation and the immune system might seem impeccable at first, it does come with a serious flaw. Inflammation can exist without any threats to the body. When this occurs, it becomes idle and loses its sense of direction. Unfortunately, inflammation is not programmed to stay inactive. In the absence of any potential invaders, it starts to damage the body instead, leading to the development of various illnesses and diseases.

In order to curb this paradox and anomaly, anti-inflammatory dietary plans work in a two-step process to reduce the risks of inflammation. Firstly, it promotes the consumption of foods that prevents inflammation. Next, it strengthens its effectiveness by eliminating other food sources that are known to support the development of inflammation. Due to the drastic change in food choices, the anti-inflammatory diet is more likely to attract people who are adaptable towards a wide variety of cuisines. For those who abstain from spicy food and fishes, or prefer to indulge in butter, cream and potatoes, an anti-inflammatory diet might not be the ideal choice.

Thanks again for downloading this book, I hope you enjoy it!

Chapter 1: Understanding Anti-Inflammatory Diet

Causes of Inflammation

The concept of an anti-inflammatory diet is relatively straightforward and the common saying of "Prevention is better than cure" can be aptly applied here. It aims to identify the origin of the problem, evaluate the options and adopt safety measures to eliminate these sources. Applying this proposition to the anti-inflammatory diet, it simply means to avoid food sources that promote the progress of inflammation while consuming more alternative food choices that are healthier with known capabilities of preventing the development of inflammation.

In general, foods that contain high levels of sugar or saturated fats possess the ability to antagonize inflammation, overloading the immune system with warnings and inadvertently causing fatigue, joint pains or even sustaining damage to the blood vessels. However, local infections are not caused by food intake only; they can be caused by other factors such as:

- High levels of stress or anxiety
- Physical Inactivity
- Vulnerability to toxins
- Genetic predisposition

Risks of Chronic Inflammation

The concept of inflammation can be medically categorized into two distinct definitions: Acute inflammation and chronic inflammation. Acute inflammation is characterized by its short-term effects that subside after a couple of days. Common occurrences of acute inflammation include:

- Infected ingrown nail
- Sprained ankle
- Sore throat
- Cuts on the skin
- Tonsillitis / Appendicitis

- Bronchitis

In contrast, chronic inflammation holds a lasting effect on the human body, primarily due to the effects of prolonged wear and tear. Environmental or habitual factors such as excess weight, physical inactivity, unhealthy diet, stress, pollution, poor oral hygiene, and excessive smoking or alcohol consumption are all known contributors to chronic inflammation. These factors can lead to a compromised health system and cause the onset of conditions such as:

- Osteoarthritis
- Lupus
- Rheumatoid Arthritis
- Asthma
- Inflammatory Bowel Disease
- Crohn's Disease
- Other Allergies

Health experts explain that the main objective of an anti-inflammatory diet is to help patients regain control of their chronic inflammation condition. While the health implications of chronic inflammation are still being explored by scientists, it has already been medically associated with several other serious conditions.

Heart Disease

The association between chronic inflammation and cardiovascular diseases has been scientifically proven by many world-renown health institutes. It should be noted that inflammation has not been proven to directly cause a heart disease or stroke. Health experts explain that inflammation only presents itself as a common element in patients who are suffering from heart conditions, and it does not necessarily indicate that the inflammation is the cause of developing these health disorders.

The inciting event of most heart attacks and strokes is the congestion of cholesterol-rich, fatty plaque in blood vessels. As the body detects this component as a foreign object that does not belong to healthy blood vessels, it reacts by engaging the plaque and actively eliminates it from the blood flow. However, this interaction between the body and the plaque can lead to blockages and blood clots in the blood vessel, consequently resulting in the onset of a heart attack or stroke. A blocked artery to the heart causes a heart attack while a blocked artery to the brain leads to an ischemic stroke.

Diabetes

The linked between chronic inflammation and diabetes was highlighted by the Clinical Division of Endocrinology and Metabolism, Department of Medicine III, Medical University of Vienna, Austria. Published in 2009, the medical literature aimed to accurately identify the association between insulin resistance, obesity, and chronic inflammation.

It explains that cytokines interference with the normal functions of insulin signaling can result in an increased insulin resistance and causes an exponential spike in sugar level. This ultimately leads to inflammation and the vicious cycle develops. Unfortunately, individuals living through this development also experiences a higher risk of excessive weight gain which can open the body to a host of diseases or disorders in the future.

Lung Issues

Asthma, chronic obstructive pulmonary disease (COPD), and infections are some of the common lung issues associated with inflammation. The Lovelace Respiratory Research Institute explains that under normal circumstances, adequate inflammation is essential to protect the lungs from pathogenic infections. When the inflammation level crosses the line to become excessive, it inevitably results in lung issues. Scientists further elaborate that airway mucus plays a vital role in the lungs' defense by immobilizing or eradicating invading pathogens. In the presence of inflammation, excessive airway mucus production inadvertently increases the risk of asthma, COPD, and even cystic fibrosis.

Bone Health

Another worrying health effect of inflammation is the compromised bone structure. Cytokines in the blood negatively influence the bone remodeling cycle, obstructing the process by which the body changes old and damaged bones with newer and healthier replacements. This subsequently leads to an increased bone resorption, a decreased bone formation, and increases bone loss. Moreover, bone health can be further impacted by inflammation to the gut as it is unable to absorb vital nutrients and minerals, such as vitamin D and calcium, that are essential for building stronger bone structures.

Depression

One of the latest developments regarding inflammation is the discovery of its effects on the mental aspects. While most medical studies have explored the physical impact of inflammation, the Centre For Addiction and Mental Health (CAMH) adopted an unusual strategy towards this issue.

Having recently released its findings in the JAMA Psychiatry Journal, the senior author points out that patients who were clinically diagnosed with depression recorded an increased brain inflammation by up to 30%. Unlike previous studies that have identified markers of inflammation in the blood, this study is the first to unearth definitive evidence of inflammation in the brain.

The study included 20 patients diagnosed with depression but who were otherwise declared healthy and 20 healthy control participants. A brain imaging technique called positron emission tomography (PET) was conducted on each of these participants. By comparing the results between all of the participants, it became clearly evident that the degree of brain inflammation increases with the development of depression. Patients with severe depression recorded the highest rates of inflammation in the brain while the healthy participants exhibited the lowest statistics.

Although this landmark discovery is still in its initial stages and might require the backing of more investigative studies, it does provide a valuable insight into the complex mental condition of depression. Other than increasing public awareness of the potential dangers of inflammation, it also paves the way for scientists to develop more potent medications that can effectively help to combat against depression.

Anger Disorders

An unlikely link between inflammation and anger issues was also discovered by researchers in 2013. The study consisted of 198 participants, with 70 of them diagnosed with an intermittent explosive disorder (IED), 61 diagnosed with other psychiatric disorders unrelated to aggression, and the 67 remaining participants with no psychiatric history served as a control.

Typical IED is characterized by repeated episodes of temper tandrums and impulsive aggression, mostly exhibited in situations such as road rage, domestic violence, or a general destructive behavior towards objects. Published by the JAMA Psychiatry Journal in 2013, the results indicate a direct correlation between inflammatory markers and symptoms of impulsive aggression. However, the scientists were unable to conclude the relationship between these two factors. It remains unclear if inflammation leads to an increased risk of aggressive behavior or if mental aggression sets off a chain reaction that leads to inflammation.

Although the study does not believe that anti-inflammatory treatments can help to reduce aggressive symptoms, it does serve as a poignant reminder of the dangers of inflammation. Coincidentally, the study provides that people suffering from IEDs also face an increased risk of heart disease, stroke, and diabetes, all of which have been directly associated with inflammation.

Test for Chronic Inflammation

In modern society, there is a heavy reliance on technology that borderlines on the edge of addiction. The extensive use of the internet has also seen many people self-diagnosing signs and symptoms of their illnesses based on information found on websites of questionable reputation. While there are no laws in place that prohibits such practices, individuals are highly recommended to seek professional advice when it comes to matters related to health.

Inflammation is a subjective and personal topic that most people would prefer to keep close to their hearts. Additionally, each individual has a different threshold for pain and the degree of pain experienced can vary drastically. The complexity of this impairment makes it difficult for people to self-diagnose simply based on information found on the internet.

Rather than referring to unregulated advice, it is more prudent to consult a doctor and receive a definite diagnosis of the problem. One of the methods to test for chronic inflammation is through the High-Sensitivity C-Reactive Protein test (hs-CRP). Elevated C-Reactive protein levels is a clear indication of inflammation and provides a reliable gauge towards the risk of future heart issues.

The process of recommending hs-CRP tests as a reliable inflammatory marker only originated in 1998. Due to the lack of a universal medical strategy to measure markers of inflammation, the American Heart Association convened the Prevention Conference V to directly address this pressing issue. In the preceding years of this landmark conference, a large number of peer-reviewed scientific reports related to inflammatory markers were published. These reports served as a reference guideline for health professionals to test for inflammation. However, the sheer volume of different tests means that there is still no general consensus within the medical field to use a uniform test to determine the presence of inflammation.

In March 2002, the CDC/AHA Workshop on Inflammatory Markers and Cardiovascular Disease: Applications to Clinical and Public Health Practice was convened to address these issues and set a reliable precedent. Through professional discussion, valuable input from the various participants and the presentation of medical evidence, it was unanimously agreed that hs-CRP tests be adopted as a reasonable measure for inflammatory markers. While the medical experts do not recommend implementing a mandatory public screening for the entire adult population, they strongly advocate that their esteemed colleagues practice discretion professional discretion in recommending this test to their patients. The need for hs-CRP tests is further enhanced in patients who exhibit higher risk factors that could indicate their susceptibility to chronic inflammation.

In the immediate aftermath of this monumental decision, other health professionals started exploring the concept of hs-CRP tests to determine its association with inflammation and other forms of diseases or disorders. In 2003, the Center for Cardiovascular Disease Prevention, Brigham and Women's Hospital, Harvard Medical School, Boston, Massachusetts, United States of America published its own review that supported the reliability of using hs-CRP measures as an inflammatory marker. Based on the health data extracted from 27,939 healthy women, it was also discovered that other than its primary function, hs-CRP is also positively correlated to the following:

- Cardiovascular disease risk
- Stronger predictor of risk compared to LDL cholesterol
- Accurately predict risk even in the absence of overt hyperlipidemia

The study further elaborates that when combined with the medical results concluded from the male population, hs-CRP presents itself as a persuasive screening alternative for patients who fall into the high-risk population. It also addresses the specific treatment of statin for inflammation, pointing out that this form of treatment is most likely to benefit patients with elevated hs-CRP levels.

Despite the serious implications of elevated hs-CRP levels, the decision to be tested for chronic inflammation ultimately rests solely on the individual, people who belong to the high-risk group are encouraged to consult with a health professional with regards to their chances of inflammation. In general, people who are at an increased risk of suffering from chronic inflammation include:

- Family history of chronic inflammation
- High cholesterol levels (Above 200)
- High blood pressure (Higher than 140/90)
- Resistant to insulin
- Diabetes
- Autoimmune diseases

People who are approaching 60 years of age are also generally more susceptible to chronic inflammation. This is due to their weakened body condition and they should consult with their personal doctors to determine if they need to be screened for chronic inflammation.

Principles of Anti-Inflammatory Diet

Each anti-inflammatory diet revolves around the idea of using food to counteract chronic inflammation that leads to serious diseases. Based on scientific knowledge of the benefits that each food offers, this form of diet is able to prevent the onset of chronic inflammation and at the same time, it serves as a general blueprint towards a healthy diet.

The main objective of an anti-inflammatory diet is to achieve and maintain optimal health condition throughout an individual's lifespan and reduce the risk of age-related diseases. One of its most distinctive traits that differentiate it from another dietary plan is the fact that it advocates the diet as a whole rather than promoting the benefits of individual foods.

As with all other forms of healthy diets, the importance of achieving a balanced variety cannot be underestimated. It is one of the prerequisites towards achieving a successful implementation of an anti-inflammatory diet. Through the inclusion of a wide variety of food choices, it ensures that the body fully absorbs all the vital nutrients and minerals that it requires to function at an enhanced capability while at the same time experience the benefits these anti-inflammatory foods.

Furthermore, health experts are quick to point out that while a healthy weight loss is an inevitable byproduct of an anti-inflammatory diet, it must not be implemented as a solution towards this objective. The primary aim of this diet is to offer relief towards inflammation and would require a prolonged period of time before visible results can be seen. However, through strict discipline and an unwavering determination, individuals who adhere to the principles of an anti-inflammatory diet will not only confer anti-inflammatory benefits, but will also help to increase energy levels and ensure the absorption of essential nutrients, vitamins, and minerals to the body.

Mechanisms of Anti-Inflammatory Diet

The prevalence of chronic inflammation for people above 60 years of age is the main reason behind many serious diseases. During healthier periods, the normal inflammation system is only activated when it senses an injury or invasion by foreign elements. As a direct consequence of the natural aging process, inflammation in a weakened body takes on another destructive persona and starts to target normal healthy tissues.

As mentioned above, this process plays a causative part in the onset of heart problems and other diseases such as Alzheimer's and Parkinson's. In order to counteract this imbalance in the body, an anti-inflammatory diet is formulated in such a way that it helps to restore the normal body function and reduce the role of potentially harmful inflammation. This is achieved through utilizing food groups that offers healthier benefits in the areas of fatty acids, carbohydrates, and fats.

A direct consequence of a more hectic lifestyle has seen most people take to fast foods and snacks as a substitute for the standard meals. These people unknowingly consume more omega-6 fatty acids than their body requires. This omega-6 fatty acids overload directly results in a higher risk of inflammation. On the other hand, omega-3 fatty acids are widely known for its anti-inflammatory effect. They are mostly found in fishes and walnuts. An anti-inflammatory diet incorporates this principle into its formulation and limits the intake of high omega-6 fatty acids while increasing consumption of omega-3 fatty acids, effectively reducing the risks of inflammation. Other ingredients that advocate inflammation are eliminated from dietary plans as well, such as hydrogenated vegetable oils and margarine.

Next, food with excess carbohydrate content indirectly endorses the inflammatory process. Consumption of these foods causes a chemical reaction between protein and sugar which in turn produces Advanced Glycation End (AGE) products. These compounds actively promote inflammation. To eliminate the production of AGE products, a stable and sufficient level of blood sugar should be monitored. This can be achieved by eating less bread, chips, processed food and fast food. Healthier alternatives are available in the form of vegetables, beans and fruits. A general preference for temperate fruits including apples, pears, berries and cherries is recommended. Tropical fruits such as bananas, mango and pineapple should be avoided.

Lastly, it is also advisable to abstain from meat and poultry due to their strong correlation to inflammation. Vegetable proteins are a healthier choice and can be derived from beans, legumes and lentils. Whole grains and nuts are also preferred while fishes such as herring, sardines, salmon and black cod are equally capable of providing the necessary protein.

Chapter 2: The Manuscript

Overview

The anti-inflammatory diet is not suitable for everyone due to the radical change in food choices and individuals might need more time to adjust to it. Furthermore, this form of diet tests the limits of an individual as it requires strict adherence over an extended period of time before noticeable results can be seen. The extensive range of food alternatives also means that there are countless ways to modify an anti-inflammatory diet. Nonetheless, a generic guideline can be applied in the formulation process to ensure that the necessary nutrients and other beneficial elements are included.

The key to developing a successful anti-inflammatory diet lies in the effective choice of food. Variety is the fundamental component as it provides the diet with an array of food choices coupled with a comprehensive coverage of benefits. A heavy favoritism towards fresh foods is important while all forms of processed food or fast food should be excluded. Fruits and vegetables should also highlight each meal based on merit as they can offer the body with loads of nutrients.

Guidelines of Anti-Inflammatory Diet

Calories

When it comes to formulating dietary plans, the first topic that comes to mind is calories. It is one of the main suspects when it comes to dealing with health issues such as weight loss. The prescribed daily intake ranges between 2000 to 3000 calories. This recommendation should be adjusted based on personal characteristics such as physical size and the amount of physical activities undertaken. People who are physically smaller or less active require a smaller intake of calories while giants and sports enthusiasts are required to consume more calories due to their heightened body requirements.

With sufficient and stable calorie intake, individual weight remains constant as well. A balanced meal should divide the intake of calories based on the proportions of 40% to 50% carbohydrates, 30% fat, and 20% to 30% proteins.

Carbohydrates

The required daily intake of carbohydrates varies across both genders. Men need roughly 300 grams on a daily basis while women, who are smaller in size, only require approximately 200 grams. Carbohydrates should be derived from food sources that are less processed and less refined as they contain a lower glycemic load.

Normal sugar and wheat products, including bread, crackers and pretzels, should be avoided. Healthier alternatives come in the form of whole grain foods, including bulgur, cereal, and rice. Other healthier sources of carbohydrates include beans, sweet potatoes, and pasta al dente. Food products that are made with fructose corn syrup should be eliminated from the diet as well.

Fat

Based on a regular 2000 calorie diet, the recommended fat content should not exceed 600 calories or 67 grams. In addition, the fat division should be in the ratio of 1 unit saturated fat to 2 units of monounsaturated fat to 1 unit of polyunsaturated fat. While this strict proportion might be too technical for the general population, individuals are advised to lay off foods such as:

- Butter
- Cream
- Unskinned chicken
- Fatty meats
- Margarine
- High-fat cheese
- Hydrogenated oil
- Vegetable shortening

Although the list might disqualify a number of food choices, there are always other better options to choose from. The benefits of avocados and nuts are strongly backed by health professionals, especially almonds, cashews, walnuts, and nut butter. Health activists also advocate the use of extra virgin olive oil. Expeller-pressed organic canola oil, sunflower oil or safflower oil can also be used instead to retain the taste of the dish. Salmon, black cod, and sardines are also suitable sources of food to satisfy the required daily intake of omega-3 fatty acids.

Other food choices include flaxseeds, hemp seeds, and omega-3 fortified eggs. For people who have distaste towards fish, fish oil supplements can take taken as an alternative but it must be ensured that EPA and DHA are both provided for. These supplements must also be molecularly distilled and labeled as free of heavy metals or other contaminants. A daily dosage of 2 grams to 3 grams is sufficient enough for the body.

Protein

Referring to a 2000 calories daily diet, protein should only occupy 80 to 120 grams of the diet. Individuals who have preexisting health conditions such as autoimmune diseases, allergies, compromised liver or kidney functions should reduce and monitor their protein consumption closely.

For the general population, animal protein should not be consumed on a regular basis, except for proteins derived from fishes. Vegetable proteins are a healthier option and it can be absorbed through eating beans, high-quality cheese or yogurts. In order to determine the suitable sources of protein based on individual preferences, it would be prudent to conduct a little trial and error in order to establish a personal list of favorites.

Fiber

Another important element in a healthy diet is the amount of fiber included. Adequate fiber consumption can be achieved through eating more whole grain products, fruits, and vegetables. Fortunately, ready-made cereals offer itself as a convenient solution towards meeting the daily fiber requirement. As a general rule of thumb, scout for reliable cereals that provides 4 to 5 grams of bran for each ounce of serving.

Phytonutrients

The main idea is to include as many different colors of foods as possible, ranging from berries to oranges to tomatoes to lemon and leafy greens. The array of benefits that come along with these foods provide the best essential protection against the common age-related diseases such as cancer, neurodegenerative disease and heart deficiencies and it is also useful in warding off the ever-present environmental toxins.

Naturally, organic products are preferred and a little personal research is required to avoid foods that contain pesticide residue. Other than a colorful plate of food, cruciferous vegetables, and soy foods should be given priority as well. In terms of beverages, reduce the consumption of coffee and switch to tea instead. Oolong, green or white tea are known to be exceptionally beneficial to the body. If alcohol consumption is preferred, red wine is the recommended choice while dark chocolate presents itself as a suitable snack in between meals.

Minerals and Vitamins

Without a doubt, the best way to load the body with minerals, vitamins and nutrients is through a hearty meal of fresh foods with a heavy dose of vegetables and fruits. In this aspect of a dietary plan, the requirements of the body can be quite complicating.

The daily supply of these nutrients can be accounted for in the form of health supplements in the following dosage:

- 2,000 IU of Vitamin D
- 800 milligrams or 400 IU of Vitamin E
- 400 milligrams of Vitamin C
- 10,000 to 15,000 IU of Mixed Carotenoids
- 200 micrograms of Selenium
- 400 micrograms of folic acid

It should be noted that there should be no additional supplement of iron except for women who are experiencing regular menstruation. Calcium supplements in the form of calcium citrate weighing 500 to 700 milligrams are also recommended for women. Across the board, vitamin A in the form of retinol should be avoided.

Water

Dietary plans often neglect to mention the benefits of water and fail to preach about the dangers of soft drinks and other concoctions. Not only are these drinks severely lacking in providing any benefits to the body, but most of them are also capable of causing internal damage as well. In a way, individuals who prefer soft drinks are literally poisoning themselves.

The anti-inflammatory diet advocates the habit of drinking pure water. In areas where chlorine or other contaminants are present in water sources, bottled water is sufficient or an adequate filter should be used. While the bland taste of pure water can ruin a sumptuous meal, alternative beverages such as lemon sparkling water, tea, and fruit juices can be used to provide variety to the table. These drinks share the same characteristic of high water content. In addition, red wine can be incorporated into certain meals as it contains the resveratrol compound that boasts anti-inflammatory properties.

Chapter 3: Foods to Avoid

The education journey towards an anti-inflammatory diet works in a two-fold process. Being knowledgeable in the requirements of this dietary plan is only the first step. To complete the course, one must also be insightful in the trigger foods that actively promote chronic inflammation. Without eliminating these sources of inflammation, no amount of anti-inflammatory food is capable of eradicating the symptoms of chronic inflammation. While different food can affect various individuals differently, the main culprits of chronic inflammation can be summarized as:

Dairy

All dairy products and milk contain a compound called casein. In most body systems, casein acts as a pro-inflammatory element and consumption should be avoided. An increasing number of people are also being diagnosed as lactose intolerant, the body's inability to digest this form of sugar. Dairy products, such as cheese, butter, and yogurt, are generally loaded with high content of casein and lactose. While total avoidance might not be possible, health experts highly recommend reduced frequency of consumption.

Wheat Products

Bread, pasta, and cookies are perfect examples of wheat products. They contain the gluten ingredient which many people are sensitive towards as they promote inflammatory. For people who are unsure whether they are vulnerable to gluten, an easy way to test is to swear off wheat products for 2 months. If they experience a significantly improved health condition, it might be an indication of high sensitivity towards gluten. Notably, the harmful effects of gluten have gained much publicity in the public media and many food products have modified their ingredient lists to offer gluten-free alternatives.

Eggs

Eggs are one of the most common ingredients in many recipes and the exclusion of it might prove to be too cumbersome. An easy workaround to this problem is to consume omega-3 fortified eggs instead to ensure that the body is able to gather nutrients from it as well. Nonetheless, some people have been discovered to be allergic to either egg whites, egg yolks or both and have to avoid eating eggs in general.

Meat

Unfortunately, meat products are only categorized as vegetable-fed or corn-fed. Producers are not required to label their meat products as organic or inorganic. However, kosher organic meat products are becoming more popular as the healthy lifestyle movement continues to establish itself. The underlying reason that advocates the abstinence of inorganic meat is due to the presence of arachidonic acid. This element is deeply embedded in the cells and initiates the PGE2 pathway, which triggers inflammation. While meat products are loved by many food enthusiasts, it might be a good time to consider the risks involved and switch to healthier options instead.

Processed Foods

Practically all processed foods are overloaded with corn syrup and sugar. Examples of these foods include candies, sweets, hot dogs and meats. Naturally, all variety of fast foods fall under this category and the occasional indulgence can be forgiven but regular reliance on them is highly frown upon by the body system.

Chapter 4: Anti-Inflammatory Foods

The factors involved in the prevalence of chronic inflammation have been established while the application of an anti-inflammatory diet has also been scientifically proven to curb the risks of inflammation within in the body. The next step of the process is to identify all types of food that are effective in preventing or curing inflammation. This will serve as the blueprint for a lifelong journey towards attaining optimum health condition.

Given the wide range of foods that are capable of warding off chronic inflammation, it might require exceptional mental strength to remember each one of them. To help with this dilemma, health experts have drawn up an anti-inflammatory diet pyramid to serve as a convenient visual representation. This pyramid categorizes all the foods that are helpful in the fight against inflammation and they are ranked according to their effectiveness.

This comprehensive 12-tier pyramid is an interactive educational tool used to address the issue of inflammation and offers individuals the ease of interpretation, regardless of their age. Ultimately, a picture's worth a thousand words. By following this graphical representation of an anti-inflammatory diet, individuals are able to provide their body with sufficient energy and adequate vitamins, minerals, dietary fiber, fatty acids and phytonutrients. Nonetheless, the effectiveness of this diet can only be witnessed after an extended period of time and people who are seeking quick and fast results should not prescribe to it.

Lastly, the healthy content of this dietary plan coincidentally offers weight loss benefits but it should not be treated as an effective weight loss alternative. The effect of weight loss should only be treated as an added incentive. The pyramid can be interpreted from the bottom (tier 1) to top (tier 12), with the effectiveness of each group ranked according to its corresponding tier (tier 1 is the most effective).

Tier 12 - Healthy Sweets

This theory was first presented at the 247th National Meeting & Exposition of the American Chemical Society (ACS), where scientists explained the mechanisms behind digesting dark chocolate and its inadvertent anti-inflammatory health benefits. Dark chocolate helps to keep the heart in top condition due to its cocoa content. As the body digests dark chocolate, microbes, and bacteria in the digestive tract ferment the fiber and antioxidant contents in cocoa. This fermentation process produces flavonols, a class of flavonoids, that can be readily absorbed into the bloodstream and offer protection against inflammation. It also possesses the capability to lower blood pressure by an average of 2 to 3 points. Nonetheless, healthy sweets should only be consumed sparingly to avoid other health complications.

Tier 11 - Red Wine

For those who love to indulge in alcohol, there is no better time to switch to red wine instead of beer or gin. Due to the resveratrol element found in red wine, the body is able to enjoy a reduced risk of inflammation which could potentially lead to cardiovascular diseases and stroke. Clinical trials have found that people who consume red wine regularly displayed lowered levels of inflammatory particles. They also showed a decreased content of monocytes and lymphocytes protein, both of which are pro-inflammatory elements. Further tests also revealed that these unique attributes are only evident through red wine consumption and not in other alcoholic beverages. Health professionals recommend that red wine consumption should be limited to a maximum of 2 glasses per day.

Tier 10 - Health Supplements

Fish oil supplements are a popular choice to treat inflammation due to the high content of docosahexaenoic acid (DHA) and eicosapentaenoic acid (EPA), normally associated with omega-3. These acids are commonly found in fish or shellfish and fish oil supplements utilize this specific characteristic to offer individuals with the same benefits of consuming a real fish. Large amounts of omega-3 fatty acids carry the unique ability to quell inflammation and effectively stop the development of other adverse health conditions. Based on a clinical trial conducted by the Department of Neurological Surgery, University of Pittsburgh Medical Center, Pittsburgh, the USA in 2006, 88% of the total participants expressed improvements in their arthritis condition after relying on fish oil supplements alone.

Tier 9 - Tea

Several variations of tea have gained much following in recent years, such as green tea, oolong tea, and white tea. While studies have shown that the flavonoid content in different types of tea is generally within the same range, it is the chemical composition of the flavonoids that differentiates the beneficial effects of each tea. Green tea, white tea and oolong tea share similar chemical composition of the catechins element that offers anti-inflammatory effects. On the other hand, other forms of tea such as black tea contain theaflavins and thearubigins which are essentially polymerized flavonoids and offers not assistance in warding off inflammation. Additionally, these tea options are also packed with other forms of nutrients that are advantageous towards improving health conditions. Daily consumption of 2 to 4 cups is sufficient for the body to absorb its benefits.

Tier 8 - Healthy Herbs and Spices

Ginger and Turmeric are common ingredients in Asian and Indian recipes with a proven track record of anti-inflammatory prowess. While ginger can help to reduce the degree of inflammation in intestines, it is more effective when taken in supplement form. Turmeric is the reason why curry is decked out in bright yellow. It has the unique ability to neutralize NF-kappa B, which is a protein that controls the immune system and initiates the inflammation mechanism. By effectively rendering this protein powerless, unnecessary inflammation is averted.

Next, garlic and onions have been known to boost the immune system. Garlic works similar to pain medications and helps to block any channels towards the development of inflammation. It acts as the first line of defense by preventing the slightest hint of inflammation to form. In contrast, onions are packed with anti-inflammatory elements such as quercetin and allicin. The disintegration of these elements produces sulfenic acid, which helps to fight against free radicals and ensure that no addition damage is done to the body.

Tier - 7 Other Protein

It should be noted that animal protein contains pro-inflammation properties, which is why the anti-inflammatory diet advocates the abstinence of general meat and poultry food sources. In contrast, vegetable proteins are beneficial to the body and can aid in preventing the onset of inflammation. Alternate sources of protein can be derived from food products such as high-quality cheese, skinless poultry, lean meat, yogurt and even omega-3 fortified eggs. However, these food choices should only be consumed at most twice in a week.

Tier 6 - Asian Mushrooms

The Chinese have long discovered the comprehensive health coverage of Asian mushrooms and have constantly utilized its properties to enhance their health condition. For example, the Shiitake mushroom contains anti-tumor properties and actively lowers cholesterol. Enoki and Maitake mushrooms offer identical benefits such as anti-cancer properties and helps to boost the immune system. All in all, the advantages of consuming these mushrooms means that they are suitable advocates in the fight against inflammation. Although the western cultures have yet to fully delve into its health benefits, eating Asian mushrooms for their anti-inflammatory properties is a good way to start. More significantly, there is no restriction levied on the consumption of these mushrooms as they offer no adverse effects.

The health benefits of these mushrooms have also generated much attention within the scientific community, with an extensive list of studies conducted to fully explore its benefits that can aid in the development of health supplements and treatment medications. One of the leading studies was published in 2008, where scientists were able to conduct scientific experiments based on the extracts of Shiitake mushrooms to determine its root source of anti-inflammatory benefits.

Other than crediting its effectiveness in treating inflammation, Asian mushrooms also play an influential role in Traditional Chinese Medicine. With practitioners prescribing different forms of Asian mushrooms as viable treatment for various health conditions. The Key Laboratory of Ministry of Education, Department of Pharmacology, Heilongjiang University of Chinese Medicine, China, acknowledges this distinct trait of Asian mushrooms and goes a step further to recommend further investigative studies into extracting properties of Asian mushrooms to develop anti-inflammatory drugs that can be easily administered into patients and treat inflammation almost instantaneously. If scientists are successful in this endeavor, it will prove to be a significant breakthrough in the medicinal field as patients suffering from chronic inflammation will have an alternative treatment option to aid in their unfortunate condition.

Tier 5 - Whole Soy Foods

Soy products contain isoflavones, which mirrors estrogens, and can help to lower the C-Reactive Protein levels in women. This process directly leads to a reduction in inflammation. More specifically, isoflavones were discovered to contain properties that can help to ease inflammation in bones and cardiovascular region.

Nonetheless, extra precaution should be taken to avoid heavily processed soy products as they do not offer the same benefits and are often overloaded with preservatives and additives. It might be more prudent to stick with safer choices such as tofu, edamame or simply fresh soy milk.

Tier 4 - Fish

Fish, specifically of the fatty category, contains high levels of omega-3 fatty acids that are known to fight off inflammation and counter the effects of excess omega-6 fatty acids at the same time. According to research conducted by the University of Hawaii in 2009, participants who consumed baked, steamed or boiled fish enjoyed a reduced risk of heart diseases by as much as 25%. Good sources of omega-3 fatty acids can be found in salmon, mackerel, tuna and sardines. The wide variety of choices enables dietary plans to include fish dishes several times a week.

In 2003, scientists based in Germany aimed to test the anti-inflammatory effectiveness of a fish-based diet in combating against the prevalence of rheumatoid arthritis. A total of 68 patients, each with definitive rheumatoid arthritis, were enrolled in the clinical trial. The participants were randomly split into two groups of 34, with the first group prescribed with a normal western diet while the second group were given an anti-inflammatory diet with less than 90 mg of arachidonic acid each day. In addition to these restrictions, random patients from both groups were given either omega-3 fish oil capsules or placebos for a period of 3 months, followed by an 8-week washout period between treatments. Clinical examinations and routine findings were evaluated on a monthly basis.

Throughout the course of the study, 8 participants dropped out, leaving the remaining 60 participants to complete the clinical trial. At the end of the observation period, the scientists arrived at the following conclusions. Participants who were given the anti-inflammatory diet with placebo treatment displayed a 14% decrease in swollen or tender joints. Patients who were prescribed with the western diet and placebo treatment displayed no improvements in their conditions. On the other hand, patients who were given fish oil supplements experienced a decrease in inflammatory symptoms regardless of their dietary plans. However, the effects of these supplements were magnified with the prescription of an anti-inflammatory diet.

Patients with the anti-inflammatory diet and fish oil supplements recorded a 28% decrease in tender joints and 34% decrease in swollen joints. Patients who were given the western diet supplemented by fish oil capsules only managed to record an 11% and 22% reduction in tender and swollen joints symptoms.

This study conclusively proves two theories. First, that an anti-inflammatory diet with less than 90 mg of arachidonic acid on a daily basis can help to ease inflammation and consequently treat rheumatoid arthritis. Secondly, it successfully establishes omega-3 fish oil as a viable treatment alternative for inflammation in the body. While this clinical trial prescribed to omega-3 fish oil in the form of health supplements, similar beneficial effects can also be obtained from consuming a regular fish diet such as those mentioned above.

This finding was echoed by a study published in the Oxford University Press, where the authors highlighted that increasing omega-3 fatty acids consumption can help to reduce the incidence rate of chronic diseases such as heart disease, inflammatory bowel disesase (IBD), cancer, rheumatoid arthritis, and even psychiatric or neurodegenerative illnesses.

Tier 3 - Healthy Fats

Extra virgin olive oil is the perfect proponent of healthy fats. Mediterranean diets have been lauded for their health benefits largely due to their generous usage of olive oil is almost every meal. The oleocanthal compound found in olive oil acts in a similar fashion to that of painkiller medications which make it a suitable candidate to ward of inflammation. Other substitutes for olive oil include expeller-pressed organic canola oil or expeller-pressed organic and high-oleic sunflower oil.

While the use of extra vigin olive oil has been widely accepted for its health benefits, most people are unaware of the scientific reasoning behind its anti-inflammatory prowess. According to the School of Exercise and Nutrition

Sciences, Centre for Physical Activity and Nutrition, Deakin University, Australia, extra virgin olive oil was first considered as an alternative treatment for inflammation due to the well-known adverse side effects of all anti-inflammatory drugs available on the market.

As mentioned above, the use of extra virgin olive oil is one of the most significant ingredients in a traditional Mediterrenean diet. It is able to confer anti-inflammatory benefits to its consumers mainly due to the presence of phenolic compounds, such as oleocanthal. These compounds exhibit similar anti-inflammatory properties as compared to medications such as iBuprofen, establishing its capabilities in treating inflammation effectively.

Another source of healthy fats can be found in nuts, especially walnuts, and almonds. Not only do they contain healthy fats, but they are also rich in fiber, vitamin E, and calcium. They also boast antioxidant properties that can prevent and repair any damage brought on by inflammation.

There is a whole range of scientific evidence credits the anti-inflammatory properties of nuts. Perhaps the most compelling evidence can be seen in the 2007 report published by the British Journal of Nutrition. The study was conducted by the Department of Biological Chemistry, Medical School, University of Athens, Greece, where the effects of walnut extracts were tested against alleviating symptoms of inflammation. The scientists identified the endothelial cell as an early indicator of inflammation and experimented its interaction in the presence of walnut extracts. By comparing the reaction of the endothelial cell in the presence and absence of walnut extracts, scientists were able to reach a general consensus that walnuts offer anti-atherogenic and anti-inflammatory properties largely due to its high content of ellagic acid.

Tier 2 - Whole Grains, Beans, Pasta

Whole grains are able to provide more fiber content and also reduce the levels of C-Reactive Protein, which is an indicator of inflammation in the blood. Additionally, whole grains contain significantly less sugar content. As a safety measure, it might be sensible to check that whole grain products have no added sugar content in their ingredient list.

Next, other than presenting themselves as healthier choices of carbohydrates, pasta al dente, and beans also displays a certain degree of effectiveness towards treating inflammation. Similar to whole grains, beans can help to lower C - reactive protein levels. They are also loaded with fiber and other phytonutrients that boast antioxidant and anti-inflammatory properties.

When combined with other anti-inflammatory foods like leafy greens, Pasta al dente itself becomes an anti-inflammatory powerhouse that magnifies the properties of other food but at the same time provides its own share of fiber, minerals and vitamins.

Tier 1 - Vegetables and Fruits

Throughout any anti-inflammation dietary plan, the influence of vegetables and fruits cannot be undermined. First of all, dark leafy greens are a good source of vitamin E and provide the body with adequate protection from pro-inflammatory molecules known as cytokines. The highest content of vitamin E can be derived from spinach, kale, broccoli or collard greens. As an added incentive, these vegetables, especially those from the cruciferous category, have a tremendous concentration of essential vitamins and minerals such as calcium, iron and other phytochemicals that are useful is fighting against diseases.

Next, the use of nightshade vegetables might be subject to debate. The undeniable fact remains that vegetables such as tomatoes, peppers, and squash have high quantities of antioxidant properties. Chili and cayenne are also rich in capsaicin, which effectively treats and reduces the pain brought on by inflammation. Oppositions of nightshade vegetables would argue that these vegetables are not suitable for people with existing health conditions such as rheumatoid arthritis. Therefore, personal judgment is necessary for making the decision of whether to include nightshade vegetables in the dietary plan.

Lastly, fruits play an equally important role in any anti-inflammatory diet. They are essential components of this diet due to their low fat and calorie content accompanied by the vast antioxidant composition. For examples, the berries family contains anthocyanins that give them unique characteristics in combating inflammation. Red raspberry helps to prevent arthritis from developing, blueberries provides protection against intestinal inflammation and ulcerative colitis, and strawberries can eradicate the build-up of C-Reactive Proteins in the blood.

Another role model of fruits is tart cherries. Scientists have established that they contain the highest antioxidant content out of all the foods and can effectively reduce inflammation in blood vessels by a staggering 50%. Tart cherries have been known to help professional athletes manage their threshold of pain and improve their individual performances simultaneously. The advantage of having fruits in any dietary plan is their versatility. They can be served as decorative to main dishes, used as a side dish or dessert, or even blended to create fresh fruit juices to accompany a sumptuous meal.

Chapter 5: Implementing an Anti-Inflammatory Diet

The anti-inflammatory diet bears a striking resemblance to Mediterranean cuisines due to the substantial inclusion of fish and spices. Food enthusiasts who are more accustomed to fast food diets or cuisines from other regions, an extended transitional period, is recommended for their body to adjust to the drastic change in food choices. Anxious people who rush into an anti-inflammatory diet ever so often find that their bodies reject the sudden switch, resulting in a growing aversion towards this form of dietary plan.

Rather than making wholesale changes to their dietary consumption, individuals who are new to the healthy lifestyle movement should adopt a cautious approach and make minor adjustments to their meals one at a time. The best way towards adopting the anti-inflammatory diet is to establish certain protocols to abide by. By gradually administering the food options provided by an anti-inflammatory diet, the body is able to cope and become readily receptive to the new choices of food.

Having determined that implementing an anti-inflammatory diet is no easy feat, individuals require as much help as they can get. By following this guide below, beginners can significantly increase their chances of conforming to this new dietary plan and advance in their journey towards a healthier lifestyle.

Build a strong support foundation

As with every lifestyle changes, having another companion to go through the experience would make the ride a lot smoother. This serves as a support system to help each party endure through all the cravings. It is also ideal to involve family members and close friends as they are the first point of contact. Not only do they function as a support, but they are also a great source of motivation. On an individual level, writing notes and putting them up is a great way to recharge willpower and ensures that the determination doesn't fade away.

Avoid making wholesale changes to other aspects of life

One major drawback of the anti-inflammatory diet is that it restricts most meals to be cooked and consumed at home. Restaurants are most likely to be in violation of anti-inflammatory regulations. Nonetheless, this does not mean that individuals have to sacrifice their social life just to stick to this strict regime. A quick workaround is to consume their meals at home first before heading out. When it comes absolute necessary to eat out, individuals can stick to just ordering salads. While this might raise a few eyebrows, do be open towards sharing the motivation for switching dietary plans. This allows others to share the experience and they might be more receptive to making similar changes in the future.

Take it slow

It is of utmost importance to exercise patience when changing to an anti-inflammatory diet. A suggested way is to incorporation the diet slowly into each meal. For example, consume only anti-inflammatory breakfast dishes for one week. For the second week, include lunch into the dietary plans. By the third week, the body would have become accustomed to the changes and a full conversion to the anti-inflammatory diet would be a resounding success.

Source for interesting recipes

Last but not least, keep a food diary and record all the food choices and recipes for each meal. As the food library grows, individuals are able to reflect on the recipes and make minor adjustments to cater to their personal preferences. This keeps the diet interesting and ensures a variation of food options.

Anti-Inflammatory Diet day meal plan example

To help kick start the conversion towards an anti-inflammatory diet, listed below are several meal suggestions to inspire beginners.

Breakfast

Option 1:

Toasted steel-cut oatmeal combined with yogurt and/or berries. Finish off the meal with a cup of hot tea, green or white.

Option 2:

Oatmeal drenched in skimmed milk, mixed with adequate amounts of berries, raisins, and walnuts based on personal preferences. Choice of green or white tea to accompany this meal.

Benefits:

Oatmeal contains flavonoids which are helpful towards reducing the risk of cardiovascular diseases while the antioxidant content in berries and tea help to fight free radicals in the body.

Lunch

Option 1:

Turkey sandwich with 100% whole wheat bread, dressed in tomato, redina lettuce and a slight dash of mayonnaise. Complete the meal with any choice of diluted fruit juice.

Option 2:

Tuna salad on whole grained bread accompanied by a mixed fruit smoothie with reduced sugar levels.

Benefits:

The choice of either sandwich or salad contains lesser amounts of fat. Whole grained bread provides a healthy intake of fiber while the inclusion of fruits ensures that the benefits of antioxidants are absorbed by the body.

Dinner

Option 1:

Spinach salad dressed in oranges, walnuts, and almonds. Spaghetti laced with turkey meat sauce and a side dish of apple pie specially made without butter.

Option 2:

Main dish of brown rice with baked salmon and decorated with oregano. Boiled asparagus lightly sprinkled with extra virgin olive oil. Salad comprising of red peppers, onion, avocado cubes, extra virgin olive oil, vinegar, red wine and tossed with spinach leaves.

Benefits:

Salmon is rich in omega-3 fatty acids while brown rice offers the necessary daily requirement of fiber. The use spinach or asparagus offers the benefits of phytonutrients while fruits enhance the variety and boasts various essential vitamins and minerals. Lastly, the resveratrol compound in red wine boasts anti-inflammatory characteristics.

Snacks/Desserts

It is very important to eat frequently to maintain your metabolism active, be sure to eat every three hours. This strategy helps your body to fight inflammation.

To simplify frequent eating, snacks are our best friends, eat snacks between main meals and you are doing the job.

Here are some snack examples.

Option 1:

Dark chocolate with a cup of walnuts.

Option 2:

Freshly sliced peaches with cinnamon and peanut butter.

Benefits:

Dark chocolates are known to reduce the risk of stroke and other heart diseases. Peaches can help to fight free radicals and also ward off the growth of cancer cells. Walnuts are also rich in omega-3 fatty acids and can help to repair any damage done by inflammation.

In each of the meal suggestions above, it is clearly evident that extra effort is put into ensuring that a variety of food choices is available. Options such as extra virgin olive oil, whole grain bread, and brown rice ensure that the principles of an anti-inflammatory diet are adhered to. The influential array of fruits and vegetables boasts highly nutritional content including antioxidants, flavonoids, omega-3 fatty acids while eliminating excess fat composition.

Chapter 6: Recipes

With all the theoretical knowledge, fundamental understanding and scientific basis of an anti-inflammatory dietary plan established, the final piece of the puzzle can now be put into place. Not many individuals are equipped with the relevant skills set to put this concept into practical application. Listed below are some suggested recipes for each meal of the day to cater to an anti-inflammatory diet.

Breakfast

Cherry Coconut Porridge

Rather than sticking to the traditional oatmeal breakfast, experience some degree of adventure by indulging in this hearty breakfast that combines the benefits of oats, cherries, and dark chocolate.

Ingredients:

- 1 ½ cups oats
- 4 cups coconut milk
- Coconut shavings
- 3 tablespoons cacao
- 4 tablespoons chia seed
- Fresh cherries
- Dark chocolate shavings
- Maple syrup
- A pinch of stevia.

Directions:

1. Mix oats, coconut milk, cacao, stevia and chia seeds in a saucepan and bring to boil over medium fire.
2. Once oats are cooked, pour mixture into a serving bowl and add in cherries, dark chocolate shavings, and maple syrup.

Raspberry Avocado Smoothie

While this fruit partnership might be weird at first glance, the creaminess of avocado helps to mask the tartness of raspberry to produce a surprisingly refreshing taste. Both fruits are well known anti-inflammatory food sources, providing an added punch to the beverage. The ease of preparation also allows individuals to add other fruits that are more appealing towards their taste palates.

Ingredients:

- 1 avocado
- ¾ cup orange juice
- ¾ raspberry juice
- ½ cup raspberries.

Directions:

1. Simply load all the ingredients into a fruit blender and mix until a uniform produce is achieved.
2. Ensure that the lumps are evenly blended in order to thoroughly enjoy this early morning drink.

Gingerbread Oatmeal

This breakfast menu offers the extensive benefits of oats but also come along with all the health benefits of the addition spices.

<u>Ingredients</u>:

- 4 cups water
- 1 cup oats
- 1 ½ tablespoons cinnamon
- ¼ teaspoon coriander
- 1 teaspoon cloves
- ¼ teaspoon ginger
- ¼ teaspoon allspice
- ¼ teaspoon cardamom
- A dash of ground nutmeg
- Maple syrup.

<u>Directions</u>:

1. Cook the oats as per normal but add in all the spices as well.
2. Once ready for consumption, add in maple syrup to taste.

Ginger Granola

For people who love granola, this breakfast option is not to be missed. This versatile breakfast dish can be consumed as a dish itself or can be accompanied by yogurt and fresh berries.

Ingredients:

- 2 cups oats
- 1 cup sunflower seeds
- 1 cup pumpkin seeds
- 1 ½ cups pitted dates
- 1 cup apple sauce
- 6 tablespoons coconut oil
- 4 tablespoons cacao and ginger.

Directions:

- Preheat oven to 356 degrees Fahrenheit
- Stir the oats and all the seeds together in a large bowl
- On the side, cook the dates in coconut oil and apple sauce until it becomes soft
- Next, peel and grate the ginger before mixing it with the dates
- Once the dates soften pour the mixture into a blender and mix it with cacao until it becomes totally smooth
- Combine both mixtures together and stir evenly
- Finally, bake the granola in the oven for 45 minutes. Throughout the baking process, stir and mix the granola every 10 minutes to ensure a balanced texture.

Crepes (Gluten-Free)

Crepes are firm breakfast favorites of many people but the normal recipe does not adhere to healthy proportions. By cooking up delicious gluten-free crepes, this breakfast choice is able to reinvent itself.

Ingredients:

- 2 eggs
- 1 teaspoon gluten-free vanilla
- ½ cup milk
- ½ cup water
- ¼ teaspoon salt
- 1 tablespoons agave nectar
- 1 cup gluten-free flour
- 2 tablespoons melted coconut oil
- 1 tablespoon coconut oil.

Directions:

1. Whisk together vanilla, eggs, milk, salt, water and agave nectar until they are evenly combined.
2. Next, add in flour slowly until both compounds merge.
3. Pour the melted coconut oil into this mixture and stir until they merge again.
4. Once completed, heat a large frying pan and set fire strength to medium.
5. Pour in batter and cook crepe for 2 minutes before flipping to cook the other side.
6. Continue the same process with the remaining batter.

Organic Vanilla Millet Muffin

This interesting organic recipe offers a slightly sweet taste that is similar to corn bread muffins but offers a distinctly higher nutritional value. Preparation takes a short 5 minutes while cooking time does not exceed 15 minutes, making this recipe an ideal breakfast choice.

Ingredients:

- 1 egg
- ¼ cup organic coconut oil, melted
- ½ teaspoon organic vanilla extract
- 1 ½ cups organic millet, cooked
- 1/3 cup turbinado sugar
- 1 teaspoon baking powder

Directions:

- Preheat oven to 350 degree Fahrenheit.
- Next, lightly grease a muffin tin.
- Combine the cooked millet, organic turbinado sugar, and baking powder into a blender and mix. If using an electric blender, ensure that the settings are adjusted to medium speed.
- Next, slowly add in egg mixture into the blender.
- Blend until a uniform paste is achieved and a smooth batter is formed.
- Scoop the batter into a prepared muffin tin and bake in the preheated oven for approximately 30 minutes.
- When the muffins have turned lightly brown, remove to a rack and allow to cool slightly
- Best served when warm.

Chocolate-Blueberry Smoothie

For those who are not keen on vanilla flavored muffins, an attractive option comes in the form of chocolate-blueberry smoothie. This delicious and gluten-free recipe is the perfect meal to kick start the day with. It can be easily prepared with ingredients found in the kitchen and the recipe can be altered slightly based on individual preferences, such as adding in other berries, dark leafy greens, or different sources of protein.

Ingredients:

- 2 tablespoons cashew
- 12 ounces water
- ½ cup frozen blueberries
- ¼ avocado
- 2 tablespoons cocoa powder
- ½ teaspoon vanilla extract
- Bee pollen

Directions:

1. Mix all ingredients into a blender and allow it to mix at a high speed setting.
2. Allow ingredients to mix for approximately 60 seconds.
3. Ensure that a uniform mixture is achieved and all ingredients are sufficiently blended.
4. Next, pour and enjoy this delicious smoothie before heading out.

Lunch

Tuna Salad

Salads present themselves as a fresh and light alternative to the other normal lunch choices. They are also easy to cook with minimal preparation time and can be served with whole grain bread or eaten by themselves.

Ingredients:

- 2 cans of tuna
- ¼ cup mayonnaise
- ¼ cup mixed olives
- 2 tablespoons minced red onion
- 2 tablespoons red peppers
- 2 tablespoons fresh basil
- 1 tablespoon capers
- 1 tablespoon lemon juice
- 2 tomatoes.

Directions:

1. Mix all ingredients, except the tomatoes, in a large bowl and stir to ensure that they are evenly spread out.
2. Pour into a serving bowl and add in the tomatoes in slices.

Red Lentil and Squash Curry Stew

This unconventional dish can be easily cooked up using any leftovers from the previous day. The ingredients are interchangeable to suit personal preferences. Nonetheless, it is packed with essential nutrients and vitamins that benefit the body.

Ingredients:

- 1 teaspoon extra virgin olive oil
- 1 chopped sweet onion
- 3 minced garlic cloves
- 1 tablespoon curry powder
- 4 cups of broth
- 1 cup red lentils
- 3 cups cooked butternut squash
- 1 cup leafy greens of choice
- 1 grated ginger.

Directions:

1. Mix olive oil, onion and garlic into a large pot and heat for 5 minutes over medium fire.
2. Next, add in curry powder, broth, and lentils.
3. Allow mixture to boil first before reducing heat.
4. Add in butternut squash and any leafy greens.
5. Cook for 5 to 8 minutes and add in seasoning to enhance the taste.

Kale Caesar Salad with Grilled Chicken Wrap

The main highlight of this dish is the use of kale. Grilled chicken is used to complement the vegetable but healthier options such as salmon can be used instead.

Ingredients:

- Grilled chicken
- 6 cups kale
- 1 cup cherry tomatoes
- ¾ parmesan cheese
- ½ egg
- 1 clove garlic
- ½ teaspoon Dijon mustard
- 1 teaspoon honey
- Sprinkles of lemon juice and olive oil
- 2 large tortillas or whole grain bread.

Directions:

1. Mix egg, garlic, mustard, lemon juice, olive oil and honey together in a bowl,
2. Add in kale, chicken and cherry tomatoes.
3. Toss thoroughly to ensure coating is balanced out.
4. Add in parmesan cheese and lay onto tortillas.
5. Roll up the wraps and serve accordingly.

Winter Fruit Salad

When in doubt, always stick to salad. This meal choice is tried and tested to provide extensive health benefits largely due to the high vegetables and fruits content.

Ingredients:

- 4 persimmons
- 3 pears
- 1 cup grapes
- ¾ cup pecans
- Extra virgin olive oil
- Vinegar and agave nectar.

Directions:

1. Mix extra virgin olive oil, vinegar, and agave nectar to formulate the dressing.
2. Cut the fruits according and toss in together with the dressing. Stir thoroughly to ensure an even spread.
3. Right before serving, add in the pecan pieces to further enhance the taste.

Roasted Red Pepper and Sweet Potato Soup

The combination of red peppers and sweet potatoes not only serves up a delightful meal, but it is also loaded with essential nutrients that are effective in fighting against inflammation.

Ingredients:

- Olive oil
- 2 chopped onions
- 12 OZ roasted and chopped red peppers
- 2 teaspoons cumin
- 1 teaspoon salt
- 1 teaspoon ground coriander
- 4 cups sweet potatoes
- 4 cup vegetable broth
- 2 tablespoons fresh cilantro
- 1 tablespoon lemon juice.

Directions:

1. Heat olive oil and cook onion until it turns soft.
2. Add in red peppers, cumin, coriander, and salt.
3. Cook slightly for a couple of minutes.
4. Add in sweet potatoes and vegetable broth
5. Allow mixture to come to a boil before decreasing heat strength and cover.
6. Season with salt to taste.

Salmon Chowder

The flavorful and anti-inflammatory profile of this dish guarantees an unforgettable taste that can rival a similar dish served in restaurants. Unlike commercial menus, the Salmon Chowder does not contain any additive, promising a fulfilled satiation at the end of the meal.

Point to take note when choosing salmon, avoid those that show hints of bruising or browning. Look for salmon with clear eyes and firm flesh that are caught in a sustainable fishery.

Ingredients:

- 1 tablespoon extra-virgin coconut oil
- ½ onion, diced
- 2 garlic cloves, chopped
- 1 celery stalk, diced
- ½ teaspoon curry powder
- 1 litre chicken stock
- 250 ml additive-free coconut milk
- 2 turnips
- Celtic sea salt
- Freshly cracked black pepper
- Fresh flat-leaf parsley
- 4 salmon fillets (skin and bones removed)

Directions:

1. Melt half of the coconut oil in a big frying pan over medium heat.
2. Add in salmon fillet and cook for 3 minutes on each side. Side aside until the fillet have cooled off sufficiently to handle. Next, flake into pieces.
3. Melt the remaining coconut oil in a large saucepan over medium heat. Add in onion, celery, garlic, curry powder, stock, turnip, and parsley. Cook for approximately 25 minutes until the onion is translucent and the turnip turns soft.
4. Next, add in 250 ml of cocounut milk and stir thoroughly to ensure both combines in a uniform fashion. Remove from heat and allow to cool.

5. Lastly, transfer both the fillets and coconut milk to puree until smooth.

Dinner

Lemon Herb Salmon

The preparations of this dish are strictly restricted to a single pan yet the flavor and nutritional values are not compromised in the cooking process.

Ingredients:

- 2 tablespoons brown sugar
- 2 tablespoons fresh lemon juice
- 1 tablespoon Dijon mustard
- 2 garlic cloves
- ½ teaspoon dried dill
- ½ teaspoon oregano
- ¼ teaspoon dried thyme
- ¼ teaspoon dried rosemary
- 4 salmon fillets
- Parsley leaves.

Directions:

1. Preheat oven to 400 degrees Fahrenheit.
2. Whisk brown sugar, lemon juice, Dijon, garlic, thyme, dill, rosemary and oregano together.
3. Next, brush each salmon with herb mixture and heat in the oven for 20 minutes.
4. Serve up with sprinkles of parsley at the side.

Stuffed Red Peppers

Not many people will think of this dish for their dinner requirements. As the name suggests the recipe centers on red peppers and is accompanied by a lean ground turkey. It offers a comprehensive range of health benefits specifically in the anti-inflammation department.

Ingredients:

- Lean ground turkey
- 3 red bell peppers
- 2 cups spaghetti sauce
- 1 teaspoon basil seasoning
- 1 teaspoon garlic powder
- ½ cup spinach
- 2 tablespoons grated parmesan cheese.

Directions:

1. Preheat oven to 450 degrees Fahrenheit.
2. Wash red bell peppers and remove the stem.
3. Split red peppers and empty the ribs and seeds inside.
4. In the meantime, dice the turkey meat and cook over medium heat.
5. Add in sauce and seasonings, cook until turkey is ready.
6. Add in spinach and parmesan cheese and stir until an evenly balanced mixture is produced.
7. Scoop turkey into the red bell peppers and decorate with sprinkles of parmesan cheese.
8. Bake for roughly 25 minutes before serving.

Baked Tilapia

Not many people would know what a tilapia is, let alone be aware of the recipe. This special fish dish incorporates the properties of brown sugar and cayenne pepper to bring about a delicious meal.

Ingredients:

- ¼ cup pecans
- ¼ cup panko breadcrumbs
- 2 teaspoon rosemary
- ½ teaspoon brown sugar
- 1 pinch cayenne pepper
- Olive oil
- 1 egg white
- 4 tilapia fillets.

Directions:

1. Preheat oven to 350 degrees Fahrenheit.
2. Mix pecans, breadcrumbs, brown sugar and cayenne pepper together.
3. Next, add in olive oil and continue to toss.
4. Bake the mixture for 7 minutes.
5. Increase oven heat to 400 degrees Fahrenheit.
6. Whisk egg white before dipping in the tilapia fillet.
7. Next, coat the fillet with the pecan mixture.
8. Bake the tilapia for roughly 10 minutes and transfer to a serving plate before consumption.

Salmon with Stone Fruit and Lavender Chutney

Salmon is a popular choice in anti-inflammatory recipes. It can be easily prepared in a variety of ways and can also be consumed at any time of the day.

Ingredients:

- 2 stone fruits
- 1 onion
- 1 lemon
- 2 tablespoons garlic
- ¼ cup red wine vinegar
- ¾ cup agave
- 2 tablespoon lavender
- Salmon.

Directions:

1. Combine all the ingredients, except the herbs, in a saucepan and bring to a boil.
2. Stir the mixture occasionally.
3. Add in the herbs and lavender after 15 minutes.
4. Next, spread the chutney atop the poached salmon and decorate with asparagus on the side.

Jolly Good Butter Chicken

An anti-inflammatory diet does not only revolve around the different types of food choices. Herbs and spices are also known to contain similar properties that can help to treat the effects of inflammation in the body. The use of these ingredients can be an important element that gives the dish a much-needed variety and help to keep the journey as interesting as possible. One of the popular dishes that utilizes herbs and spices is the Jolly Good Butter Chicken, guaranteed to satisfy the taste buds while offering essential anti-inflammatory benefits.

Ingredients:

- 1 tablespoon sesame oil
- 1 kg free-range chicken breast, thickly sliced
- 70 g unsalted butter
- 1 teaspoon garam masala
- 1 cinnamon stick
- 10 cardamon pods
- 1 teaspoon sweet paprika
- 1 teaspoon ground cumin
- 1 teaspoon ground chilli
- 400 g tinned diced tomatoes
- 1 tablespoon sugar and additive-free tomato paste
- 400 ml additive-free coconut milk
- 370 g steamed brown rice
- 1 Lebanese cucumber, diced and chilled
- 1 ripe banana, sliced
- 1 teaspoon shredded coconut
- 1 dollop of mango chutney

Directions:

1. Add sesame oil to a large saucepan over high heat.
2. Divide the chicken into 2 batches to cook, each for a period of 5 minutes or cook till it turns brown.
3. Set aside each batch while cooking the remaining chicken.
4. Remove both batches of chicken once cooked.
5. Reduce heat on the saucepan and add in butter.

6. Add in all the spices, stir and cook for approximately 5 minutes until the fragrance is fully extracted.
7. Added in the both batches of chicken, together with tomato paste and tomatoes.
8. Stir and simmer for 20 minutes.
9. Turn down the heat to low settings and add in the coconut milk.
10. Simmer for 5 minutes.
11. Mix the banana and coconut in a small bowl.
12. Best served with brown rice with saffron, turmeric, and cucumber salad.

CONCLUSION

Thank you again for downloading this book!

I hope this book was able to help you to understand the fundamental concept of an anti-inflammatory diet and the mechanics behind this form of dietary plan that makes it one of the most effective methods towards an improved health condition.

The next step is to start putting the knowledge to good use and protect yourself against the threat of chronic inflammation. Bear in mind the principles of the 12 tiered pyramid and fully utilize the full variety of foods to achieve an interesting dietary plan based on your personal taste. If you are unsure of where to start, take inspiration from the suggested recipes and feel free to modify the ingredients list to better suit your digestive system.

Finally, if you enjoyed this book, then I'd like to ask you for a favor, would you be kind enough to leave a review for this book on Amazon? It'd be greatly appreciated!

Click here to leave a review for this book on Amazon!

Thank you and good luck!

www.ingramcontent.com/pod-product-compliance
Lightning Source LLC
LaVergne TN
LVHW090823151224
799147LV00042B/1288